I0223285

100 Stress Reducing Meal and Juice Recipes:

Get Through Tough Times and Moments of Anxiety by Eating Delicious Foods

By

Joe Correa CSN

COPYRIGHT

© 2018 Live Stronger Faster Inc.

All rights reserved

Reproduction or translation of any part of this work beyond that permitted by section 107 or 108 of the 1976 United States Copyright Act without the permission of the copyright owner is unlawful.

This publication is designed to provide accurate and authoritative information in regard to the subject matter covered. It is sold with the understanding that neither the author nor the publisher is engaged in rendering medical advice. If medical advice or assistance is needed, consult with a doctor. This book is considered a guide and should not be used in any way detrimental to your health. Consult with a physician before starting this nutritional plan to make sure it's right for you.

ACKNOWLEDGEMENTS

This book is dedicated to my friends and family that have had mild or serious illnesses so that you may find a solution and make the necessary changes in your life.

100 Stress Reducing Meal and Juice Recipes:

Get Through Tough Times and Moments of Anxiety by Eating Delicious Foods

By

Joe Correa CSN

CONTENTS

ABOUT THE AUTHOR

After years of Research, I honestly believe in the positive effects that proper nutrition can have over the body and mind. My knowledge and experience has helped me live healthier throughout the years and which I have shared with family and friends. The more you know about eating and drinking healthier, the sooner you will want to change your life and eating habits.

Nutrition is a key part in the process of being healthy and living longer so get started today. The first step is the most important and the most significant.

INTRODUCTION

100 Stress Reducing Meal and Juice Recipes: Get Through Tough Times and Moments of Anxiety by Eating Delicious Foods

By Joe Correa CSN

Eliminating all the factors that cause stress is almost impossible. However, the best way to boost your energy and leave stress behind is starting a healthy diet! This is a no-brainer. A healthy diet will balance your entire body in a way that you can't even imagine. A balanced diet will stabilize your blood sugar levels and give you enough energy to deal with a stressful situation and emotional issues in the best possible manner.

This is exactly why I have created this book with healthy and great-tasting recipes that focus on increasing fiber and good carbs to keep blood sugar levels in check. These recipes are full of natural sources of all kinds of nutrients your body so desperately needs in order to deal with everyday life. Fruits and vegetables, legumes, beans, healthy lean meats, lots of salmon and olive oil, nuts and seeds. There is absolutely nothing better than eating smarter to lower stress levels.

I have prepared these delicious meal and juice recipes for stress that you can make at home. I have combined some of the best stress combating fruits and vegetables in powerful mixes that should assist you in dealing with stress.

There is something for all taste buds and I hope these carefully selected and tried recipes will help you lead the stress free existence you deserve.

A proper, balanced diet full of these precious nutrients helps not only deal with stress and binge eating but will affect your entire life and health.

Stop living a life of stress by preparing these tasty meal and juice recipes daily. Make them part of your life!

100 STRESS REDUCING MEAL AND JUICE RECIPES

Meals

1.   Pasta with Arugula Sauce

Ingredients:

2 lbs of pasta, pre-cooked

2 cups of fresh arugula, trimmed

1 cup of cream cheese

2 tsp of lemon juice, freshly squeezed

4 garlic cloves, minced

2 tbsp of pine nuts, toasted

½ tsp of salt

Preparation:

Cook pasta using package instructions. Drain well and set aside.

Meanwhile, combine cheese, arugula, lemon juice, garlic, and salt in a food processor. Blend until nicely smooth. Pour the sauce over the pasta and top with pine nuts.

Serve.

Nutrition information per serving: Kcal: 595, Protein: 20.7g, Carbs: 85.1g, Fats: 19.0g

2.   Salmon with Salsa Potatoes

Ingredients:

2 lbs of wild salmon filets, skinless and boneless

1 tbsp of olive oil

1 tbsp of rosemary, finely chopped

½ tsp of sea salt

4 small potatoes, peeled and chopped

For the salsa:

2 medium-sized tomatoes, diced

1 small onion, diced

¼ cup of fresh parsley, chopped

1 tbsp of lemon juice

1 tsp of apple cider vinegar

½ tsp of salt

Preparation:

Place the potatoes in a pot of boiling water. Cook until fork-tender. Remove from the heat and drain. Transfer to a serving plate and set aside.

Combine all salsa ingredients in a food processor and blend until smooth. Transfer to a bowl and set aside.

Preheat the oil on a large nonstick pan over a medium-high temperature. Add meat and cook for about 4-5 minutes, or until set. Transfer the meat to a serving plate with potatoes. Sprinkle the meat with rosemary and salt. Pour the salsa over the potatoes and serve.

Nutrition information per serving: Kcal: 235, Protein: 23.9g, Carbs: 15.8g, Fats: 9.0g

3.   Avocado Chutney

Ingredients:

2 large avocados, pitted, peeled, and chopped

1 medium-sized onion, diced

1 tsp of fresh ginger, grated

1 tsp of cumin, ground

½ cup of fresh mint, finely chopped

1 tbsp of olive oil

½ tsp of salt

¼ tsp of black pepper, ground

Preparation:

Preheat the oil in a large skillet over a medium-high temperature. Add onions and stir-fry until translucent. Stir in cumin and ginger and cook for about 3-4 minutes more. Remove the skillet from the heat and stir in avocado and mint.

Sprinkle with some salt and pepper to taste and serve.

Nutrition information per serving: Kcal: 340, Protein: 3.6g, Carbs: 17.1g, Fats: 31.2g

4.   Basmati Rice

Ingredients:

3 cups of basmati rice

2 small red onions, diced

1 cup of spring onions, chopped

1 large bell pepper, chopped

1 medium-sized carrot, chopped

3 tbsp of lemon juice

1 tbsp of balsamic vinegar

1 tsp of curry powder

½ tsp of Cayenne pepper, ground

½ tsp of salt

¼ tsp of black pepper, ground

Preparation:

Mix together lemon juice, vinegar, curry, Cayenne pepper, salt, and pepper in a mixing bowl. Set aside to allow flavors to mingle.

Place the rice in a deep pot. Pour 6 cups of water and bring it to a boil. Now, reduce the heat to low and cover with a lid. Cook for 40 minutes, or until tender. Remove from the heat and drain. Set aside.

Meanwhile, combine red onions, spring onions, and carrot in a large bowl. Drizzle with lemon juice mixture and stir well. Add rice and mix all to combine.

Serve.

Nutrition information per serving: Kcal: 440, Protein: 9.1g, Carbs: 96.4g, Fats: 1.0g

5.   Orange Beet Salad

Ingredients:

2 large oranges, peeled and wedged

5 medium-sized beets, trimmed, peeled

2 cups of Romaine lettuce, chopped

2 cups of black beans, pre-cooked

1 tbsp of red wine vinegar

3 tbsp of fresh dill, minced

2 tbsp of extra-virgin olive oil

2 tbsp of almonds, roughly chopped

½ tsp of salt

¼ tsp of black pepper, ground

Preparation:

Mix together vinegar, oil, dill, salt, and pepper in a mixing bowl. Set aside.

Place the beets in a deep pot and add water enough to cover it. Bring it to a boil then reduce the heat. Cover with a lid and cook for about 20-25 minutes, or until fork-tender. Remove from the heat and drain well. Set aside.

Meanwhile, place the beans in a pot of boiling water. Cook until soften, then remove and drain well. Set aside.

Now, combine beets, beans, and oranges in a large bowl. Drizzle with dressing and toss well to coat.

Place a handful of lettuce on a serving plate and spoon the beet salad. Top with almonds and sprinkle with salt and pepper, if needed.

Nutrition information per serving: Kcal: 345, Protein: 16.8g, Carbs: 57.8g, Fats: 6.9g

6.   Zucchini Cream Soup

Ingredients:

4 medium-sized zucchinis, peeled and chopped

1 medium-sized onion, chopped

2 cups of vegetable broth

1 cup of plain yogurt

1 tsp of dried thyme, minced

1 tsp of nutmeg

1 tsp of lime zest

½ tsp of black pepper, ground

½ tsp of salt

Preparation:

Combine onions and 2 tablespoons of water in a large nonstick skillet over a medium-high temperature. Add zucchinis and cook for 5 minutes stirring constantly. Pour the vegetable stock and stir in nutmeg, thyme, and lime zest.

Cook for another 15 minutes, or until fork-tender. Remove from the heat and transfer to a food processor.

Blend until nicely smooth, then return to the skillet. Stir in the yogurt and heat it up. Sprinkle with salt and pepper if needed and serve.

Nutrition information per serving: Kcal: 63, Protein: 5.0g, Carbs: 8.3g, Fats: 1.2g

7.   Cucumber Tuna Wraps

Ingredients:

4 cans of tuna, drained

2 medium-sized cucumbers, chopped

½ cup of shallots, finely chopped

4 tbsp of mayonnaise

¼ cup of lemon juice

2 tbsp of sour cream

½ tsp of salt

¼ tsp of black pepper, ground

1 large lettuce head

Preparation:

Mix together mayonnaise, lemon juice, sour cream, and a pinch of salt in a small bowl. Set aside.

Combine tuna, shallots, cucumber in a large bowl. Stir in the previously made mixture and toss to mix well with a spoon.

Spread the lettuce leaves on a serving plate and spoon the mixture. Wrap and secure with a toothpick. Serve immediately.

Nutrition information per serving: Kcal: 253, Protein: 28.1g, Carbs: 7.4g, Fats: 11.9g

8.   Vegetable Hash

Ingredients:

2 cups of white beans, pre-cooked

½ cup of leeks, finely chopped

1 large bell pepper, finely chopped

2 small potatoes, peeled and chopped

1 cup of fresh kale, chopped

2 garlic cloves, minced

2 tsp of fresh rosemary, finely chopped

2 tbsp of lemon juice

1 tbsp of lemon zest

1 tsp of salt

½ tsp of black pepper, ground

Preparation:

Place potatoes in a pot of boiling water. Cook until soften and remove from the heat. Drain well and set aside. Repeat the process with beans.

Combine leeks, pepper and 2 tablespoons of water in a large nonstick saucepan over a medium-high temperature. Cook for 2 minutes, then add garlic. Sprinkle with rosemary and stir well. Add potatoes, lemon juice, and beans. Cook for about 8-10 minutes then add kale. Cook for another 5 minutes, or until kale soften. Sprinkle with lemon zest, salt, and pepper before serving.

Nutrition information per serving: Kcal: 342, Protein: 21.0g, Carbs: 65.1g, Fats: 1.0g

9.   Gingerbread Cookies

Ingredients:

2 cups of whole-wheat flour

1 tsp of baking soda

1 tsp of ginger, ground

1 tsp of cinnamon, ground

½ cup of applesauce

2 tbsp of maple syrup

2 tbsp of fig jam

1 tsp of vanilla extract

Preparation:

Preheat the oven to 375°F.

Combine flour, baking soda, cinnamon, ginger, and vanilla. Stir well then add maple syrup, applesauce, and fig jam. Mix until you get a nice batter. Form the cookies in desired size or shape.

Place a baking paper over a large baking sheet. Spread the cookies with 2 inches of space in between. Bake for 5-6 minutes, or until crispy browned. Remove from the oven and let it cool for a while.

Serve with honey or milk. This is, however, optional.

Nutrition information per serving: Kcal: 91, Protein: 2.2g, Carbs: 19.6g, Fats: 0.2g

10. Juicy Beef & Green Beans

Ingredients:

2 lbs of lean beef, cut into bite-sized pieces

2 large bell pepper, seeded and stripped

4 garlic cloves, minced

½ cup of fresh dill, finely chopped

2 cups of green beans, pre-cooked

3 tbsp of olive oil

1 tbsp of lemon juice

¼ tsp of Cayenne pepper, ground

½ tsp of salt

¼ tsp of black pepper, ground

Preparation:

Preheat the oven to 375°F.

Combine bell peppers, 2 tablespoons of oil, garlic, dill, lemon juice, cayenne pepper, salt, and pepper in a food processor. Blend until smooth and set aside.

Place the green beans in a pot of boiling water and cook until fork-tender. remove from the heat and drain well. Set aside.

Preheat the remaining oil in a large skillet over a medium-high temperature. Add meat and sprinkle with salt and pepper to taste. Cook for 10 minutes, or until golden brown. Remove from the heat and transfer to a serving plate with green beans. Drizzle with dressing and serve.

Nutrition information per serving: Kcal: 379, Protein: 47.9g, Carbs: 8.7g, Fats: 16.8g

11.   Cooked Red Cabbage and Apples

Ingredients:

1 large red cabbage head, shredded

2 medium-sized carrots, diced

1 cup of fresh celery, diced

2 medium-sized apples, peeled, cored and chopped

1 medium-sized onion, diced

2 tbsp of yellow mustard

4 tbsp of red wine vinegar

2 tbsp of olive oil

1 tsp of dried thyme, ground

½ tsp of salt

¼ tsp of black pepper, ground

Preparation:

Preheat the oil in a large nonstick skillet over a medium-high temperature. Add onions and stir-fry for a few minutes until translucent. Add celery, carrots, about 2 tablespoons of water, thyme, vinegar, and mustard. Cook for 5 minutes, stirring occasionally.

Add apples and cabbage and reduce the heat to low. Cover with a lid and cook for 20 minutes, or until tender.

Sprinkle with salt and pepper to taste before serving.

Nutrition information per serving: Kcal: 133, Protein: 2.5g, Carbs: 21.9g, Fats: 5.2g

12.   Oven-Baked Creamy Turkey Avocado

Ingredients:

4 lbs of turkey breasts, thinly sliced

1 medium-sized avocado, pitted, peeled, and chopped

1 large bell pepper, chopped

1 cup of Parmesan cheese, shredded

2 tbsp of fresh parsley, finely chopped

2 tbsp of Dijon mustard

½ cup of corn, kernel removed

4 tbsp of butter

½ tsp of Himalayan salt

Preparation:

Preheat the oven to 375°F.

Coat the meat with mustard in a large bowl. Set aside.

Melt the butter in a nonstick skillet over a medium-high temperature. Add avocado, pepper, cheese, parsley, and corn. Stir and cook until cheese is melted. Remove from the heat and transfer the mixture to a large baking dish. Add meat and coat with mixture. Cover the dish with aluminum foil and put it in the oven.

Bake for 45 minutes, or until heated trough. Remove from the oven and let it cool for a while before serving.

Nutrition information per serving: Kcal: 315, Protein: 35.1g, Carbs: 12.3g, Fats: 13.9g

13.   Garlic Meatballs

Ingredients:

1lb lean beef, minced

7 oz of white rice

2 small onions, peeled and finely chopped

2 garlic cloves, crushed

1 large egg, beaten

1 large potato, peeled and sliced

3 tbsp of extra-virgin olive oil

1 tsp of salt

Preparation:

In a large bowl, combine lean ground beef with rice, finely chopped onions, crushed garlic, one beaten egg, and salt. Shape the mixture into 15-20 meatballs, depending on the size.

Grease the bottom of your slow cooker with three tablespoons of olive oil. Make the first layer with sliced potatoes and top with meatballs.

Cover, set the heat to low and cook for 6-8 hours.

Nutrition information per serving: Kcal: 468, Protein: 33.4g, Carbs: 47.0g, Fats: 15.3g

14.   Peanut Butter Chicken

Ingredients:

4 lbs of chicken filets, thinly sliced

4 tbsp of peanut butter

1 cup of skim milk

¼ cup of fresh cilantro, finely chopped

4 tbsp of vegetable oil

4 tsp of ginger, ground

1 tbsp of sea salt

¼ tsp of black pepper, ground

Preparation:

Preheat the oven to 400°F.

Place the meat in a large baking dish and coat with sea salt. Set aside.

Preheat the oil in a large nonstick saucepan over a medium-high temperature. Add milk, cilantro, and ginger. Cook for 2 minutes then stir in ginger and pepper. Cook for another 2 minutes then add peanut butter. Stir well to combine and cook for another minute. Remove from the heat.

Pour the peanut butter mixture over the meat. Cover with a lid and place it in the oven. Bake for about 15-20 minutes, or until golden brown. Remove the lid and bake for 2 more minutes. Remove from the oven and let it cool for a while before serving.

Nutrition information per serving: Kcal: 371, Protein: 55.1g, Carbs: 3.0g, Fats: 14.2g

15.   Choco-Berry Smoothie

Ingredients:

1 cup of fresh strawberries

1 cup of frozen raspberries

5 egg whites

½ cup of coconut milk

¼ cup of chocolate chips

1 tbsp of honey

1 tbsp of flaxseed

Preparation:

Combine strawberries, raspberries, egg whites, coconut milk, and chocolate chips in a food processor. Blend until nicely smooth. Add water to adjust the thickness. Add honey and re-blend. Transfer the mixture to a serving glasses and top with flaxseeds for extra taste and nutrients.

Enjoy!

Nutrition information per serving: Kcal: 330, Protein: 9.3g, Carbs: 42.9g, Fats: 14.8g

16.   Toasted Nuts

Ingredients:

½ cup of almonds

½ cup of pistachios

½ cup of cashews

½ cup of walnuts

4 tbsp of butter

1 tsp of nutmeg

1 tsp of orange zest

1 tsp of cinnamon, ground

1 tsp of ginger, ground

1 tsp of salt

Preparation:

Preheat the oven to 350°F.

Combine all nuts in a large bowl.

Place some baking paper on a large baking dish and spread the nuts. Put it in the oven and roast for about 8-10 minutes. Remove from the oven and set aside to cool for a while.

Melt the butter in a large nonstick frying pan over a medium-high temperature. Add cinnamon, nutmeg, ginger,salt, and orange zest. Stir well to combine and add nuts. Cook 1 minute and remove from the heat.

Serve immediately.

Nutrition information per serving: Kcal: 412, Protein: 10.6g, Carbs: 12.9g, Fats: 38.4g

17.   Creamy Lemon Salmon with Spinach

Ingredients:

2 lbs of wild salmon filets, thinly sliced

4 cups of spinach, finely chopped

1 cup of coconut milk

½ cup of lemon juice

1 tbsp of lemon zest

4 tbsp of fresh parsley, finely chopped

2 tbsp of pine nuts

2 tbsp of olive oil

1 tsp of salt

¼ tsp of black pepper, freshly ground

Preparation:

Preheat 1 tablespoon of oil in a large nonstick skillet over a medium-high temperature. Add meat and sprinkle with some salt to taste. Cook for 5 minutes on each side, or until golden brown. Set aside

Preheat the remaining oil in a separate frying pan and add spinach. Cook until slightly soften. Stir in pine nuts and cook for 1 minute more. Remove from the heat and transfer to a serving plate. Top with salmon and set aside.

Combine coconut milk and lemon juice in a medium saucepan. Heat it up and pour over the meat. Sprinkle with lemon zest before serving.

Nutrition information per serving: Kcal: 363, Protein: 31.5g, Carbs: 4.2g, Fats: 25.8g

18.   Chocolate Orange Yogurt

Ingredients:

1 cup of plain yogurt, or Greek yogurt

¼ cup of dark chocolate, grated

1 large orange, peeled and wedged

1 tbsp of honey

1 tbsp of chia seeds

A few mint leaves

Preparation:

Combine yogurt and chia in a medium bowl. Stir in the honey and mix well with a spoon.

Add grated chocolate and orange. Mix well and sprinkle with some fresh mint to taste.

Nutrition information per serving: Kcal: 268, Protein: 12.9g, Carbs: 36.0g, Fats: 9.6g

19.   Veal Steak in Garlic and Red Pepper Sauce

Ingredients:

1 lb of veal steak, boneless

3 large bell peppers, chopped

3 tbsp. of olive oil

4 cloves of garlic, chopped

1 small onion, chopped

1 tsp. of dried rosemary, finely chopped

½ cup of water

Non-fat cooking spray

Preparation:

Preheat oven to 350°F.

Lightly coat a baking sheet with cooking spray. Place the meat on a baking sheet and cook for 60 minutes.

Meanwhile, cut each pepper in half, remove the stem and seeds. Finely chop your peppers. Heat up the olive oil in a saucepan and add garlic and onion. Saute until translucent. This should take no more than 5 minutes. Stir constantly. Add peppers, rosemary and ½ cup of water (you can add some more water if the sauce is too thick). Bring it to a boil and reduce the heat to minimum. Cook for 10-15 minutes. Set aside.

When the meat is nice and tender, remove from the oven and transfer to a plate. Pour the pepper sauce over the meat chops and serve.

Nutrition information per serving: Kcal: 258, Protein: 46.0g, Carbs: 17.2g, Fats: 18.3g

20.   Eggplant and Ground Beef Casserole

Ingredients:

2 large eggplants, thinly sliced

1 cup of lean beef, ground

1 medium-sized onion, chopped

1 tsp of olive oil

¼ tsp of black pepper, freshly ground

2 medium-sized tomatoes, cubed

3 tbsp of fresh parsley, finely chopped

Preparation:

Preheat the oven to 300°F.

Peel the eggplants and cut lengthwise into thin sheets. Put them in a bowl, and leave them to sit for at least an hour. Roll them in beaten eggs.

Preheat the oil in a large skillet over a medium-high temperature. Add eggplants and fry for 3 minutes on each side, or until set. Set aside.

Preheat the remaining oil in the same skillet. Stir-fry the onions until translucent, then add, tomato, and sprinkle with pepper and parsley. Cook for 2 minutes and add meat. Cook until tender.

Remove from the heat and set aside to cool for a while.

Combine meat and vegetable mixture and egg in an ovenproof dish and spread on the bottom. Make one layer with eggplants, then again meat and veggies. Repeat the process with remaining ingredients.

Bake for 30 minutes or until doneness. Remove from the oven and serve.

Nutrition information per serving: Kcal: 114, Protein: 14.2g, Carbs: 21.6g, Fats: 9.7g

21. Coco Vanilla Smoothie

Ingredients:

1 cup of coconut milk

½ cup of water

1 tsp of vanilla extract

1 tsp of vanilla, ground

¼ cup of fresh raspberries

½ cup of fresh strawberries

¼ tsp of cinnamon, ground

Preparation:

Combine milk and water in a deep pot. bring it to a boil on a low temperature. Add vanilla and vanilla extract. Stir well and let it boil for about a minute. Remove from the heat and allow it to cool.

Combine milk mixture with all other ingredients in a blender. Blend until smooth and transfer to a serving. Refrigerate for 1 hour before serving.

Nutrition information per serving: Kcal: 79, Protein: 4.6g, Carbs: 10.2g, Fats: 1.6g

22.   Sweet Swedish Salmon

Ingredients:

2 medium-sized salmon fillets, boneless

1 tsp of cumin, ground

1 tbsp of olive oil

1 tsp of lime juice

1 tsp of cinnamon, ground

1 tsp of paprika, ground

½ tsp salt

¼ tsp of black pepper, ground

Preparation:

Preheat the oven to 350°F.

Combine lime juice, cinnamon, paprika, salt, and pepper in a mixing bowl.

Place the salmon into the mixture and coat well. Cover with plastic wrap and place in the fridge. Marinade for 30 minutes in the refrigerator.

Now place the salmon pieces onto a greased baking tray. Bake for nearly 6-8 minutes and serve hot.

Nutrition information per serving: Kcal: 117, Protein: 18.2g, Carbs: 12.6g, Fats: 8.3g

23.   Mexi-Pulled Beef

Ingredients:

3 lbs lean beef roast

½ cup apple cider vinegar

1 tbsp of vegetable oil

1 tsp of salt

2 tbsp of dried onions, chopped

1 tbsp of cumin, ground

3 tbsp of onion powder

1 garlic clove, minced

3 tbsp of chili powder

Preparation:

Combine cumin, onion, garlic, chili, and salt in a mixing bowl. Set aside to allow flavors to mingle.

With a cooker's lid off, preheat the oil over a medium-high temperature. Add onions and stir-fry for 5 minutes.

Meanwhile coat and rub the meat with the mixture of spices. Place the beef roast in the cooker and cook for about 10-12 minutes, or until browned.

Now add the remaining ingredients and securely lock the pressure cooker's lid. Set for 8 minutes on high.

Perform a quick release to release the cooker's pressure.

Nutrition information per serving: Kcal: 135, Protein: 15.62g, Carbs: 5.4g, Fats: 8.3g

24.   Fresh Frisee with Walnuts

Ingredients:

1 lb of frisee lettuce, trimmed and roughly torn

¼ cup of walnuts

1 small Honeycrisp apple, cored

¼ cup of champagne vinegar

3 tsp of yellow mustard

½ cup of extra-virgin olive oil

¼ tsp of salt

¼ tsp of black pepper, ground

Preparation:

Combine champagne vinegar, mustard, olive oil, salt, and pepper in a blender. Blend well to combine. Set aside.

Trim and roughly torn the frisee in a bowl. Slice the apple into thin matchsticks. Stir in the walnut and drizzle with blended mixture. Toss well to combine. Serve cold.

Nutrition information per serving: Kcal: 315, Protein: 2.7g, Carbs: 12.3g, Fats: 30.3g

25.   Shrimp Skewers Salad with Lemon Chili Dressing

Ingredients:

For the grilled shrimps and tomatoes:

5 large shrimps, peeled and deveined

8 oz grape tomatoes

1 tbsp of olive oil

2 garlic cloves, crushed

1 tsp of fresh cilantro, minced

½ tsp of turmeric, ground

1 tsp of salt

¼ tsp of black pepper, ground

2 skewers, soaked in water

For the salad:

½ head butter lettuce, roughly chopped

½ medium-sized avocado, pitted, peeled and sliced

For the dressing:

¼ cup of lemon juice, freshly squeezed

¼ cup of extra-virgin olive oil

1 tsp of yellow mustard

¼ tsp of chili powder

½ tsp of cumin, ground

1 tbsp of scallions, minced

¼ tsp of sea salt

Preparation:

Preheat an electric grill over a high temperature. Mix together 3 tablespoons of olive oil, crushed garlic, fresh cilantro, turmeric powder, salt, and pepper. Stir until completely combined.

Skewer shrimps and tomatoes and spread the marinade over it using a kitchen brush. Grill for about 2-3 minutes on each side. Remove from the grill and set aside.

Combine the dressing ingredients in a small bowl. Place the butter lettuce and avocado in a bowl. Top with shrimps and tomatoes, and drizzle with the lemon-chili dressing. Enjoy!

Nutrition information per serving: Kcal: 223, Protein: 3.1g, Carbs: 7.2g, Fats: 21.6g

26.   Tuna Steaks with Coriander and Lemon Juice

Ingredients:

¼ cup of fresh coriander, chopped

3 garlic cloves, minced

2 tbsp of lemon juice

½ cup olive oil

4 tuna steaks

½ tsp smoked paprika

½ tsp of cumin, ground

½ tsp of chili powder

½ tsp of salt

¼ tsp of black pepper, ground

Preparation:

Add the coriander, garlic, paprika, cumin, chilli powder and lemon juice in a food processor and pulse to combine. Gradually add in the oil and mix the ingredients until a smooth mixture.

Transfer the mixture into a bowl, add the fish and gently toss to coat the fish evenly with sauce. Chill for at least 2 hours to allow the flavors to penetrate into the fish.

Remove the fish from the chiller and preheat the grill. Lightly brush the grid with oil, place the fish and grill for about 3 to 4 minutes on each side.

Remove the fish from the grill, transfer to a serving plate and serve with lemon wedges or some vegetables.

Nutrition information per serving: Kcal: 513, Protein: 54.6g, Carbs: 1.2g, Fats: 31.7g

27.   Fresh Cabbage Lamb Stew

Ingredients:

3 lbs of lamb, boneless, pre-cooked

1 ½ lbs of fresh cabbage

1 large red onion, peeled and sliced

4 garlic cloves, crushed

1 large tomato, finely chopped

½ cup of parsley, finely chopped

4 tbsp of extra-virgin olive oil

6 cups of water

3 bay leaves

Preparation:

Pour 6 cups of water into the pressure pot and add the meat. Securely lock the cooker's lid and set for 10 minutes on high.

Perform a quick release to release the cooker's pressure.

Now add the vegetables and spices. Pour enough water to cover all ingredients. Securely lock the cooker's lid again and set for 25 minutes on high.

Serve warm.

Nutrition information per serving: Kcal: 401, Protein: 31.86g, Carbs: 62.13g, Fats: 5.12g

28.   Blueberry Honey Smoothie

Ingredients:

1 cup of fresh blueberries

¼ cup of almonds, toasted

1 tbsp of chia seeds

1 cup of almond milk

2 tbsp of honey, raw

A handful of ice cubes

Preparation:

Combine all ingredients in a blender. Blend until smooth and transfer to a serving glasses. Serve immediately.

Nutrition information per serving: Kcal: 225, Protein: 11.4g, Carbs: 31.3g, Fats: 8.1g

29.   Chicken Honey with Spring Onions

Ingredients:

1 lb of chicken thighs, cut into bite-sized pieces

4 tbsp of honey, raw

6 spring onions, chopped

1 tbsp of fresh mint, finely chopped

6 tsp of cinnamon, ground

1 tbsp of coconut oil

1 tsp of cumin, ground

1 tsp of black pepper, ground

1 tsp of sea salt

Preparation:

Preheat the oil in a large nonstick saucepan over a medium-sized temperature. Add meat and cook for about 8-10 minutes, or until golden brown.

Add chopped onion and toss for another 3 minutes. Add the seasoning and the cumin to it. Sprinkle the cinnamon and add the honey. Toss for 5 minutes more and check if the chicken has cooked through.

Garnish with mint and serve hot.

Nutrition information per serving: Kcal: 105, Protein: 12.9g, Carbs: 11.8g, Fats: 1.1g

30.   Fresh Coriander Soup

Ingredients:

4 cups of vegetable broth

2 green chili pepper, finely chopped

6 medium-sized tomatoes, halved

½ tsp of cumin, ground

1 red onion chopped

2 cups of fresh coriander, chopped

1 tsp of almond flour

¼ cup of fresh parsley, chopped

2 tbsp of ginger garlic paste

½ tsp of coriander, chopped

½ tsp of black pepper, ground

½ tsp of sea salt

1 tsp of almond butter

Preparation:

In a large pot, melt the almond butter and fry the chopped

red onion for nearly 3 minutes. Add the ginger garlic paste to it.

Add the pepper, salt, coriander, cumin, and green chilies. Toss for 3 minutes and then add the tomatoes. Give it a good stir and then pour in the broth.

Cook on low heat for about 1 hour. Serve hot.

Nutrition information per serving: Kcal: 115, Protein: 4.2g, Carbs: 18.6g, Fats: 5.3g

31. Roasted Lamb Chops

Ingredients:

2x 1 ½ inch-thick lamb loin chops

1 cup of vegetable oil

3 garlic cloves, crushed

1 tbsp of fresh thyme leaves, crushed

1 tbsp of fresh rosemary, crushed

1 tbsp of red pepper, ground

1 tsp of sea salt

Preparation:

Preheat the oven to 350°F.

Combine the oil with crushed garlic, thyme, rosemary, red pepper, and salt. Mix well in a large bowl. Add lamb loin chops and turn to coat. Let it stand in the refrigerator for about 2 hours.

Place the lamb chops in a large, ovenproof skillet. Add 4 tablespoons of marinade and reduce the heat to 300°F. Cook for about 15 minutes and remove from the oven. Now add remaining marinade, turn over the chops, and cook for 15 more minutes.

Remove from the oven and serve with fresh vegetables. Enjoy!

Nutrition information per serving: Calories: 411, Protein: 45.6g Carbs: 19.4g Fats: 21.2g

32. German Stew

Ingredients:

3 lbs of beef chuck shoulder, boneless

1 lb of beef marrow bones

1 large carrot, sliced

3 small onions, peeled

1 lb of button mushrooms, sliced

2 cups of beef stock

10 garlic cloves

2 tbsp of olive oil

1 tbsp of dry rosemary, ground

½ tsp of salt

¼ tsp of black pepper, ground

Preparation:

Preheat the oil in a frying skillet over a medium-high temperature. Add beef and brown on both sides. Remove from the skillet and season generously with salt and pepper.

Transfer to a pressure cooker. Add beef bones, sliced carrot, mushrooms, garlic, rosemary and beef stock.

Securely lock the lid and set to 24 minutes on high.

Perform a quick release to release the cooker's pressure. Remove the bones and serve.

Nutrition information per serving: Kcal: 370, Protein: 46.5g, Carbs: 40.2g, Fats: 29.6g

33. Sweet Corn Salad

Ingredients:

½ cup of Romaine lettuce, finely chopped

½ cup of sweet corn

1 medium-sized red bell pepper, sliced

½ medium-sized green bell pepper, sliced

5 cherry tomatoes, halved

½ red onion, peeled and sliced

1 tsp of dry rosemary, crushed

1 tsp of lime juice

Preparation:

Wash and cut the bell peppers in half. Remove the seeds and the pulp. Slice into thin slices.

Peel and slice the onion.

Use a big serving platter and arrange the vegetables. You can play with some colors, or even add some ingredients you like. Sprinkle with some rosemary and fresh lime juice. Serve immediately.

Nutrition information per serving: Kcal: 370, Protein: 46.5g, Carbs: 40.2g, Fats: 29.6g

34.   Healthy Leek Stew

Ingredients:

6 large leeks, trimmed

1 lb of lean beef

1 bay leaf

1 medium-sized carrot, sliced

¼ cup of celery, chopped

1 small onion, peeled and sliced

¼ tsp of black pepper, ground

½ tsp of salt

5 tbsp of extra-virgin olive oil

½ tsp of dry rosemary, finely chopped

Preparation:

Grease the bottom of the pressure cooker with 2 tablespoons of olive oil. Coat the meat with some salt and pepper and place in the cooking pot.

Add sliced onion, carrot, celery, and 1 bay leaf. Pour enough water to cover all ingredients and seal the lid. Bring the cooker up to full pressure and reduce to a minimum. Cook for 45 minutes. Remove from the heat and set aside.

Trim the leeks and remove the first two layers. Chop into bite-sized pieces. Heat up the olive oil over medium-high temperature and stir-fry the leeks for several minutes.

Remove the meat from the cooking pot. Chop into smaller pieces and add to the frying skillet. Add dry rosemary and some salt to taste. Cook for another 10-12 minutes.

Nutrition information per serving: Kcal: 420, Protein: 19.3g, Carbs: 25.5g, Fats: 27.4g

35.   Coconut Pudding

Ingredients:

2 cups of coconut milk

1 tbsp of walnuts, finely chopped

1 tbsp of hazelnuts, finely chopped

2 tsp of cocoa powder, raw

1 tsp of cinnamon, ground

½ tbsp of vanilla powder

1 tsp of honey

Preparation:

Pour 2 cups of milk into a deep pot and bring it to a boil.

Add nuts, cocoa, honey, vanilla, and stir well. Cook for about 10 minutes, or until you get a creamy mixture.

Stir in some cinnamon and remove from the heat. Allow it to cool in the refrigerator before serving.

Nutrition information per serving: Kcal: 140, Protein: 3.4g, Carbs: 20.6, Fats: 4.6g

36.   Italian Casserole

Ingredients:

4 large eggplants, sliced

2 medium-sized onions, peeled and chopped

10 large tomatoes, roughly chopped

7 oz green olives

7 oz capers

1 medium-sized chili pepper

2 stalks of celery, chopped

½ cup of extra-virgin olive oil

3 tbsp of apple cider vinegar

1 tsp of salt

1 tsp of honey

½ tbsp of basil, dry

Preparation:

Chop the eggplants into bite-sized pieces and season with some salt. Allow it to stand for about 30 minutes and rinse well.

Transfer to a crock pot and add other ingredients. Cover and cook for about 2 hours over a medium temperature.

It can stand in the refrigerator for a couple of days.

Nutrition information per serving: Kcal: 98, Protein: 12.3g, Carbs: 19.4g, Fats: 9.6g

37.　Baby Spinach & Apple Smoothie

Ingredients:

½ medium-sized apple, peeled and sliced

1 cup of baby spinach, finely chopped

1 cup of orange juice, freshly squeezed

2 tbsp of flaxseeds

1 tsp of honey, raw

Preparation:

Combine all ingredients except ice cubes in a blender; purée until smooth. Add ice cubes and re-blend. Transfer the mixture to serving glasses. Enjoy!

Nutrition information per serving: Kcal: 140, Protein: 7.5g, Carbs: 24.0g, Fats: 2.4g

38. Creamy Broccoli Soup with Lemon Juice

Ingredients:

2 oz of fresh broccoli, trimmed

¼ cup of fresh parsley, finely chopped

1 tsp of dried thyme, ground

1 tbsp of fresh lemon juice

¼ tsp of chili pepper, ground

3 tbsp of olive oil

1 tbsp of cashew cream

Preparation:

Place the broccoli in a deep pot and pour enough water to cover. Bring it to a boil and cook until tender. Remove from the heat and drain.

Transfer to a food processor. Add fresh parsley, thyme, and about ½ cup of water. Pulse until smooth mixture. Return to a pot and add some more water. Bring it to a boil and reduce the temperature to low. Cook for 10 minutes.

Stir in some olive oil and cashew cream, sprinkle with ground chili pepper and add fresh lemon juice. Serve warm.

Nutrition information per serving: Kcal: 72, Protein: 12.4g, Carbs: 15.8g, Fats: 8.3g

39.   Wild Salmon with Fresh Dill

Ingredients:

1 lb of wild salmon, thinly sliced

½ cup of lemon juice, freshly squeezed

1 garlic clove, crushed

1 large egg, beaten

½ tsp of sea salt

1 tbsp of dry parsley, crushed

½ cup of fresh dill, chopped

¼ cup of extra virgin olive oil

2 tbsp of olive oil

Preparation:

Preheat the oven to 350°F.

Combine the olive oil with lemon juice, crushed garlic clove, one egg, salt, and parsley. Mix well and place the salmon slices in it. Cover and marinate for about an hour.

Pour the salmon slices along with marinade in a small baking dish. Bake for 35 minutes. Remove from the oven, and sprinkle with fresh mint.

Nutrition information per serving: Kcal: 235, Protein: 27.3g, Carbs: 5.8, Fats: 9.2g

40.　　Cider Mustard Chicken Breast

Ingredients:

2 chicken breasts, boneless and skinless

¼ cup of apple cider vinegar

¼ cup of extra-virgin olive oil

2 garlic cloves, crushed

2 tbsp of yellow mustard

½ tsp of green pepper, freshly ground

2 tbsp of olive oil

Preparation:

Wash and pat dry meat. Place it on a cutting board and season with ground green pepper.

In a large bowl, combine the apple vinegar, olive oil, garlic and mustard to make a marinade. Soak the chicken breast into this marinade and make sure it all gets coated nicely. Cover and place in the refrigerator for at least 2 hours (the best option is to keep it in the refrigerator overnight).

Preheat 1 tablespoon of oil in a large skillet over a medium-high temperature. Add chicken and fry for 7-10 minutes on each side, until nice crispy and light brown. Add some of the marinade mixture while frying the chicken. These juices will make the meat soft. Stir occasionally and check if the chicken is fully cooked. Serve.

Nutrition information per serving: Kcal: 396, Protein: 33.3g, Carbs: 1.2g, Fats: 28.3g

41.   Northern Pate

Ingredients:

2 salmon filets, skinless and boneless

½ tsp of dry rosemary

1/8 tsp of sea salt

¼ tsp of chili pepper, ground

1 tbsp of fresh lemon juice

1 tbsp of extra-virgin olive oil

Preparation:

Wash and pat dry the salmon fillets. Cut into bite- sized pieces and set aside.

Heat up the olive oil in a large skillet over amedium high temperature. Add tuna chops and cook for about 10 minutes, stirring constantly. Remove from the heat and transfer to a food processor.

Add 2 tablespoons of olive oil, lemon juice, salt, chili pepper and rosemary. Process well until nicely combined. Serve with some fresh vegetables.

Nutrition information per serving: Kcal: 240, Protein: 20.2g, Carbs: 1.2g, Fats: 16.3g

42.   Fresh Mint Smoothie

Ingredients:

1 cup of chopped broccoli

¼ cup of spinach, chopped

½ cup of water

½ cup of coconut water, unsweetened

1 tbsp of walnuts, ground

A few mint leaves

Preparation:

Wash the vegetables and place into a blender. Put some ice cubes and blend together until smooth mixture.

Top with walnuts and garnish with mint leaves.

Nutrition information per serving: Kcal: 94, Protein: 4.9g, Carbs: 12g, Fats: 2.7g

43. Almond Butter Chocolate

Ingredients:

8 oz cocoa, raw

1 cup of almond butter, melted

1 cup of almond milk

¼ cup of almond flour

4 large eggs

1 cup of honey, raw

5 tbsp of almond cream

Preparation:

Preheat the oven to 300°F.

Place some baking paper over a baking dish and set aside.

Combine all dry ingredients in a large bowl and mix well to combine. Whisk in the eggs, melted almond butter, almond milk, and almond cream.

Transfer the mixture to a prepared baking dish and bake for about 30-35 minutes. Allow it to cool for 1 hour and serve.

Nutrition information per serving: Kcal: 212, Protein: 1.6g, Carbs: 31.3, Fats: 11.4g

44.   Sweet Chicken Thighs

Ingredients:

2 lbs of chicken thighs, boneless

2 medium-sized onions, chopped

2 small chili peppers, chopped

1 cup of chicken broth

¼ cup of fresh orange juice

1 tsp of organic orange extract

2 tbsp of extra-virgin olive oil

1 tsp of barbeque seasoning mix

1 small red onion, chopped

Preparation:

Preheat the oven to 350°F.

Heat up the olive oil in a large saucepan over a medium-high temperature. Add chopped onions and stir-fry for several minutes, until golden color.

Combine chili peppers, orange juice and orange extract in a food processor. Blend for 30 seconds. Add this mixture to a saucepan and stir well. Reduce heat to simmer.

Coat the chicken with barbecue seasoning mix and put it into a saucepan. Add chicken broth and bring it to a boil. Cook over a medium-high temperature until all the water evaporates. Remove from the heat.

Place the chicken into a large baking dish. Bake for about 15 minutes to get a nice crispy, golden brown color.

Nutrition information per serving: Kcal: 170, Protein: 38.5g, Carbs: 11.6g, Fats: 21.7g

45.   Vanilla Mousse

Ingredients:

½ cup of blueberries

¼ cup of strawberries

½ glass of coconut milk

2 cups of water

1 tbsp of almond cream

1 tbsp of powdered vanilla

½ tsp of cinnamon

Preparation:

Combine the ingredients in a food processor and pulse until you get a nice smooth mixture. Top with mixed nuts or seeds on your choice.

Nutrition information per serving: Kcal: 134 Protein: 11.3g, Carbs: 38.3, Fats: 15.9g

46. Cashew Cream and Avocado Puree

Ingredients:

2 large eggs

2 egg whites

1 tbsp of cashew cream

½ cup of almond milk

1 ripe avocado, pitted, peeled, and roughly chopped

1 tbsp of fresh mint leaves, finely chopped

1 tsp of salt

Preparation:

Hard boil the eggs for about 8-10 minutes. Remove from the heat and allow it to cool.

Peel and cut the eggs. Mash with a fork. Separate the egg whites from yolks.

Peel and chop avocado. Place it in a blender. Add almond milk, eggs, egg whites, cashew cream, salt, and mint leaves.

Blend well for about 30 seconds. Serve cold.

Nutrition information per serving: Kcal: 187, Protein: 12.8g, Carbs: 7.4g, Fats: 4.5g

47.   Grilled Chicken Breast with Parsley

Ingredients:

1 large chicken breasts, skinless and boneless, chopped

¼ cup of extra virgin olive oil

3 garlic cloves, crushed

½ cup of fresh parsley, chopped

1 tbsp of fresh lime juice

1 tsp of salt

Preparation:

Combine the olive oil with crushed garlic cloves, finely chopped parsley, fresh lime juice and some salt.

Wash and pat dry the meat and cut into 1-inch thick pieces. Pour the olive oil mixture over the meat and let it stand for about 15 minutes.

Preheat the grill pan over a medium-high temperature. Add 2 tablespoons of marinade in the grill pan and chicken fillets. Cook for about 15 minutes.

Remove from the pan and serve with some vegetables of your choice.

Nutrition information per serving: Kcal: 439, Protein: 44.2g, Carbs: 1.6g, Fats: 28.1g

48. Ginger Smoothie

Ingredients:

1 cup of mixed blueberries, raspberries, blackberries and strawberries

½ cup of baby spinach, chopped

½ cup of coconut milk

1 ½ cup of water

¼ tsp of ginger, ground

A handful of fresh mint leaves

Preparation:

Wash the baby spinach and combine with other ingredients in a blender. Mix well for 30 seconds. Serve immediately.

Nutrition information per serving: Kcal: 72, Protein: 6.4g, Carbs: 11.3g, Fats: 2.9g

49.   Lean Beef and Mangel Stew

Ingredients:

7 oz of lean beef

1 large red onion, chopped

4 tbsp of olive oil

½ chili pepper, sliced

3 cups of water

8 oz of mangel, diced

2 medium -sized sweet potatoes, chopped

3 oz of broccoli, trimmed

1 large carrot, chopped

1 large tomato, sliced in cubes

½ cup of tomato sauce

8 cups of water

¼ tsp of Cayenne pepper

2 tbsp of all-purpose flour

Preparation:

Preheat 2 tablespoons of oil in a pot over a medium-high temperature. Add chopped onion and fry for a few minutes, or until golden brown.

Now, add the lean beef, 4 cups of water, and a pinch of salt. Cover and leave it to cook for 15 minutes.

Remove from the heat and add prepared vegetables and tomato sauce. Add 4 more cups of water and transfer to a slow cooker.

Meanwhile, heat up the remaining oil over a medium-high temperature. Add cayenne pepper and flour and stir well. Add the mixture to the slow cooker and cook for about 2 hours. Remove from the heat and give it a good stir before serving.

Nutrition information per serving: Kcal: 295, Protein: 35.4g Carbs: 39.5g Fats: 19.3g

50. Cilantro Pork Stew

Ingredients:

8 oz of pork shoulder, cut into 1-inch thick pieces

1 small onion, sliced

1 cup of beef stock

¼ cup of water

½ cup of green tomatillo salsa

A handful of fresh cilantro, roughly chopped

1 tsp of salt

¼ tsp of black pepper, ground

Preparation:

Place the meat in a large glass bowl. Coat well with salt and pepper.

Place the meat and sliced onion in a deep pot. Pour the beef stock and bring it to a boil. Reduce the heat and add about ½ cup of water and green tomatillo salsa.

Mix well, cover and simmer for about 40 minutes, stirring occasionally.

Serve with fresh cilantro.

Nutrition information per serving: Kcal: 274 Protein: 27.3g, Carbs: 21.1g, Fats: 8.5g

Juices

1. Fennel Swiss Chard Juice

Ingredients:

3 large Granny Smith's apples, cored

1 cup of fennel, chopped

1 cup of fresh spinach, torn

1 cup of Swiss chard, torn

Preparation:

Wash the apples and cut in half. Remove the core and cut into bite-sized pieces. Set aside.

Wash the fennel bulb and trim off the wilted outer layers. Cut into small chunks and fill the measuring cup. Reserve the rest in the refrigerator.

In a large colander, combine Swiss chard and spinach. Rinse thoroughly under cold running water and drain. Torn with hands and set aside.

Now, combine fennel, Swiss chard, spinach and apple in a

juicer. Process until well juiced.

Transfer to a serving glass and refrigerate for 15 minutes before serving.

Enjoy!

Nutritional information per serving: Kcal: 220, Protein: 5.0g, Carbs: 66.3g, Fats: 1.3g

2.   Pomegranate Beet Juice

Ingredients:

1 cup of beet greens, chopped

1 cup of beets, sliced

1 cup of pomegranate seeds

1 cup of celery, chopped

1 tbsp of honey

Preparation:

Wash the beets and trim off the green parts. Cut into bite-sized pieces and set aside.

Use the trimmed beet greens and roughly chop it.

Cut the top of the pomegranate fruit using a sharp knife. Slice down to each of the white membranes inside of the fruit. Pop the seeds into a measuring cup and set aside.

Wash the celery and cut into small pieces. Set aside.

Now, process beets, beet greens, pomegranate seeds, and celery in a juicer.

Transfer to serving glasses and stir in the honey.

Add some ice and serve immediately.

Enjoy!

Nutritional information per serving: Kcal: 113, Protein: 5.1g, Carbs: 33.9g, Fats: 1.4g

3.   Blackberries Lime Juice

Ingredients:

1 cup of blackberries

1 whole lime, peeled

1 cup of pomegranate seeds

1 small Granny Smith's apple, cored

¼ tsp of ginger, ground

2 oz of water

Preparation:

Place the blackberries in a colander. Rinse well under cold running water and drain. Set aside.

Peel the lime and cut lengthwise in half. Set aside.

Cut the top of the pomegranate fruit using a sharp paring knife. Slice down to each of the white membranes inside of the fruit. Pop the seeds into a measuring cup and set aside.

Wash the apple and cut lengthwise in half. Remove the core and cut into bite-sized pieces and set aside.

Now, combine pomegranate seeds, blueberries, lime, and apple in a juicer and process until juiced. Transfer to a serving glass and stir in the ginger and water.

Refrigerate for 10 minutes before serving.

Enjoy!

Nutritional information per serving: Kcal: 206, Protein: 3.3g, Carbs: 61.1g, Fats: 1.8g

4. Orange Cucumber Juice

Ingredients:

1 cup of cucumber, sliced

1 medium-sized zucchini, chopped

1 large orange, peeled and wedged

1 cup of pumpkin, cubed

1 large carrot, sliced

1 small ginger knob, chopped

Preparation:

Wash the cucumber and cut into thin slices. Fill the measuring cup and reserve the rest for later. Set aside.

Peel the zucchini and chop into small pieces. Set aside.

Peel the orange and divide into wedges. Cut each wedge in half and set aside.

Cut the top of a pumpkin. Cut lengthwise in half and then scrape out the seeds. Cut one large wedge and peel it. Cut into small cubes and fill the measuring cup. Reserve the rest in the refrigerator.

Wash and peel the carrot. Cut into thin slices and set aside.

Peel the ginger knob and cut into small pieces. Set aside.

Now, combine pumpkin, carrot, cucumber, orange, and ginger in a juicer. Process until well juiced. Transfer to a serving glass and add some ice.

Serve immediately.

Nutrition information per serving: Kcal: 133, Protein: 5.7g, Carbs: 38.2g, Fats: 1.0g

5. Papaya Zucchini Juice

Ingredients:

1 medium-sized zucchini, chopped

1 cup of fresh basil, torn

1 cup of cucumber, sliced

1 cup of red leaf lettuce, torn

1 cup of papaya, chopped

Preparation:

Combine basil and lettuce in a large colander and rinse under cold running water. Drain and torn with hands into small pieces. Set aside.

Wash the cucumber and cut into thin slices. Fill the measuring cup and refrigerate for later.

Peel the zucchini and chop into small pieces. Set aside.

Peel the papaya and cut lengthwise in half. Scoop out the black seeds and flesh using a spoon. Cut into small chunks and set aside.

Now, combine zucchini, basil, cucumber, lettuce and papaya in a juicer. Process until well juiced. Transfer to a serving glass and add some ice.

Serve immediately.

Nutrition information per serving: Kcal: 92, Protein: 4.7g, Carbs: 25.8g, Fats: 1.3g

6.   Cauliflower Honeydew melon Juice

Ingredients:

1 cup of cauliflower, chopped

1 cup of fresh basil, torn

1 large wedge of honeydew melon

1 medium-sized red apple, cored

1 large lemon, peeled

Preparation:

Trim off the outer leaves of a cauliflower. Wash it and fill and cut into small pieces. Fill the measuring cup and reserve the rest in the refrigerator.

Wash the basil thoroughly under cold running water. Slightly drain and chop into small pieces. Set aside.

Cut the honeydew melon lengthwise in half. Scoop out the seeds using a spoon. Cut one large wedge and peel it. Cut into small chunks and place in a bowl. Wrap the rest of the melon in a plastic foil and refrigerate.

Wash the apple and cut lengthwise in half. Remove the core and cut into bite-sized pieces. Set aside.

Peel the lemon and cut lengthwise in half. Set aside.

Now, combine cauliflower, basil, honeydew melon, apple and lemon in a juicer. Process until well juiced and transfer to a serving glass.

Add few ice cubes and serve immediately.

Enjoy!

Nutritional information per serving: Kcal: 156, Protein: 9.06g, Carbs: 46.43g, Fats: 1.55g

7.   Sweet pepper Carrot Juice

Ingredients:

1 large sweet pepper, chopped

1 medium-sized cucumber, sliced

2 large carrots, sliced

1 cup of fresh basil, chopped

¼ tsp of ginger, ground

Preparation:

Wash the sweet pepper and cut lengthwise in half. Remove the stem and seeds. Cut into small pieces and set aside.

Wash the cucumber and cut into thin slices. Fill the measuring cup and refrigerate for later.

Wash and peel the carrots. Cut into thin slices and set aside.

Wash the basil thoroughly under cold running water. Slightly drain and chop into small pieces. Set aside.

Now, combine sweet pepper, cucumber, carrots, and basil, in a juicer and process until juiced. Transfer to a serving glass and stir in the ginger. Add some water if needed.

Refrigerate for 5 minutes before serving.

Nutrition information per serving: Kcal: 130, Protein: 5.9g, Carbs: 37.1 g, Fats: 1.2g

8.   Cauliflower Papaya Juice

Ingredients:

3 cauliflower flowerets, chopped

1 cup of papaya, chopped

1 large orange, peeled and wedged

1 whole lime, peeled

1 whole leek, chopped

Preparation:

Wash the cauliflower flowerets thoroughly and chop into small pieces. Set aside.

Peel the papaya and cut lengthwise in half. Scoop out the black seeds and flesh using a spoon. Cut into small chunks and set aside.

Peel the orange and divide into wedges. Cut each wedge in half and set aside

Peel the lime and cut lengthwise in half. Set aside.

Wash the leek and cut into small pieces. Set aside.

Now, combine cauliflower, avocado, lime, and leek in a juicer and process until juiced. Transfer to a serving glass and refrigerate for 10 minutes before serving.

Enjoy!

Nutritional information per serving: Kcal: 184, Protein: 4.6g, Carbs: 55.5g, Fats: 1.g

9.   Lemon Spinach Juice

Ingredients:

1 cup of spinach, torn

1 whole lemon, peeled

1 cup of blueberries

1 whole lime, peeled

1 tbsp honey, raw

2 oz of water

Preparation:

Wash the spinach thoroughly under cold running water. Slightly drain and torn into small pieces. Set aside.

Peel the lemon and lime. Cut each fruit lengthwise in half and set aside.

Rinse the blueberries using a small colander. Slightly drain and fill the measuring cup. Set aside.

Now, combine spinach, lemon, lime, and blueberries in a juicer and process until juiced. Transfer to a serving glass and stir in the water and honey.

Garnish with some mint, but it's optional.

Refrigerate for 10 minutes before serving.

Enjoy!

Nutrition information per serving: Kcal: 103, Protein: 4.5g, Carbs: 33.8g, Fats: 1g

10. Apple Kale Juice

Ingredients:

2 small Granny Smith's apple, cored

1 cup of cucumber, sliced

2 cups of fresh kale, chopped

1 large wedge of honeydew melon

1 cup of watercress, torn

1 cup of fresh parsley, torn

1 oz of water

Preparation:

Wash the apples and cut lengthwise in half. Remove the core and cut into bite-sized pieces. Set aside.

Wash the cucumber and cut into thin slices. Fill the measuring cup and reserve the rest for later. Set aside.

Wash the kale thoroughly under cold running water. Chop into small pieces and set aside.

Cut the honeydew melon lengthwise in half. Scoop out the seeds using a spoon. Cut one large wedge and peel it. Cut into small chunks and place in a bowl. Wrap the rest of the melon in a plastic foil and refrigerate.

Combine watercress and parsley in a colander. Rinse well under cold running water and torn with hands. Set aside.

Now, combine apples, cucumber, kale, and watercress, honeydew melon, and parsley in a juicer and process until juiced. Transfer to a serving glass and stir in the water. Add some ice before serving.

Enjoy!

Nutritional information per serving: Kcal: 259, Protein: 10.7g, Carbs: 71.5g, Fats: 2.5g

11.   Carrots Grapefruit Juice

Ingredients:

2 medium-sized carrots, sliced

1 large orange, peeled

1 whole grapefruit, wedged

1 whole lemon, peeled

1 small pear, cored and chopped

1 small ginger knob, peeled

Preparation:

Wash and peel the carrot. Cut into thin slices and set aside.

Peel the orange and divide into wedges. Cut each wedge in half and set aside.

Peel the grapefruit and divide into wedges. Cut each wedge in half and set aside.

Wash the pear and remove the core. Cut into bite-sized pieces and set aside.

Peel the lemon and cut lengthwise in half. Set aside.

Peel the ginger knob and set aside.

Now, combine carrots, broccoli, orange, lemon and, ginger knob in a juicer. Process until juiced.

Transfer to a serving glass and refrigerate for 15 minutes before serving.

Nutritional information per serving: Kcal: 202, Protein: 5.0, Carbs: 67.3g, Fats: 1g

12.   Artichoke Cucumber Juice

Ingredients:

1 large artichoke, head

1 whole cucumber, sliced

1 whole lime, peeled

1 large carrot, sliced

1 cup of fresh cilantro, torn

¼ tsp turmeric, ground

Preparation:

Wash the artichoke and trim off the outer leaves. Cut into small pieces and fill the measuring cup. Reserve the rest in the refrigerator.

Wash the cucumber and cut into thick slices. Set aside.

Peel the lime and cut lengthwise in half. Set aside.

Wash and peel the carrot. Cut into thin slices and set aside.

Add cilantro in a colander. Rinse well under cold running water and torn with hands. Set aside.

Now, combine artichoke, cucumber, lime, cilantro and

carrot in a juicer and process until juiced. Transfer to a serving glass and stir in the turmeric.

Refrigerate for 10 minutes before serving.

Nutrition information per serving: Kcal: 126, Protein: 9.8g, Carbs: 42.3g, Fats: 1.2g

13.   Watermelon Guava Juice

Ingredients:

1 whole grapefruit, wedged

1 large orange

1 cup of watermelon

1 large green apple, cored

1 large guava

2 oz of coconut water

Preparation:

Peel the grapefruit and divide into wedges. Cut each wedge in half and set aside.

Peel the orange and divide into wedges. Set aside.

Cut the watermelon lengthwise. For one cup, you will need about one large wedge. Peel and cut into chunks. Remove the seeds and set aside. Reserve the rest of the melon for some other juices.

Wash the apple and remove the core. Cut into bite-sized pieces and set aside.

Wash the guava and cut into chunks. If you are using large

fruit, reserve the rest for some other recipe in a refrigerator.

Now, combine grapefruit, orange, watermelon, apple, and guava. Transfer to serving glasses and stir in the coconut water.

Add some ice or refrigerate before serving.

Enjoy!

Nutritional information per serving: Kcal: 320, Protein: 6.8g, Carbs: 95.2g, Fats: 1.7g

14.   Cantaloupe Mint Juice

Ingredients:

2 cups of cantaloupe, cubed

1 whole grapefruit

1 cup of fresh mint, torn

¼ tsp of cinnamon, ground

1 oz coconut water

Preparation:

Cut the cantaloupe in half. Scoop out the seeds and flesh. Cut and peel one large wedge. Chop into chunks and fill the measuring cup. Reserve the rest of the cantaloupe in a refrigerator.

Peel the grapefruit and divide into wedges. Cut each wedge in half and set aside.

Wash the mint thoroughly and torn with hands into small pieces. Set aside.

Cut the cantaloupe in half. Scoop out the seeds and flesh. Cut and peel one large wedge. Chop into chunks and fill the measuring cup. Reserve the rest of the cantaloupe in a refrigerator.

Now, combine cantaloupe, grapefruit, and mint, in a juicer. Process until well juiced.

Transfer to a serving glass and stir in the cinnamon and coconut water. Add some ice and serve immediately.

Nutrition information per serving: Kcal: 191, Protein: 5.4g, Carbs: 55.4g, Fats: 1.1g

15. Spinach Raspberries Juice

Ingredients:

1 cup of spinach, torn

1 cup of raspberries

1 cup of cantaloupe, diced

1 cup of parsley, chopped

1 medium-sized cucumber, peeled

1 tbsp of honey, raw

Preparation:

Combine spinach and parsley in a colander and wash under cold running water. Torn with hands and set aside.

Wash the raspberries and set aside.

Cut the cantaloupe in half. Scoop out the seeds and flesh. Cut two wedges and peel them. Chop into chunks and set aside. Reserve the rest of the cantaloupe in a refrigerator.

Wash the cucumber and cut into thick slices. Set aside.

Now, process spinach, raspberries, cantaloupe, parsley, and cucumber in a juicer.

Transfer to serving glasses and stir in the honey.

Refrigerate for 10 minutes before serving.

Enjoy!

Nutritional information per serving: Kcal: 197, Protein: 10.2g, Carbs: 58.3g, Fats: 2.2g

16.   Papaya Lettuce Juice

Ingredients:

1 cup of papaya, chopped

1 cup of cabbage, torn

1 cup of red leaf lettuce, torn

2 large pears, cored

1 whole lime, peeled

1 tbsp of coconut sugar

½ cup of pure coconut water, unsweetened

Preparation:

Peel the papaya and cut lengthwise in half. Scoop out the black seeds and flesh using a spoon. Cut into small chunks and set aside.

Combine cabbage and lettuce in a colander and wash under cold running water. Torn with hands and set aside.

Wash the pears and cut lengthwise in half. Remove the core and cut into small pieces. Set aside.

Now, process papaya, cabbage, pears, lettuce, and lime in a juicer.

Transfer to serving glasses and coconut water and coconut sugar.

Add some ice and serve immediately.

Nutritional information per serving: Kcal: 285, Protein: 4.2g, Carbs: 96.1g, Fats: 1.2g

17.   Celery Cauliflower Juice

Ingredients:

1 cup of celery, chopped

1 cup of cauliflower, chopped

1 large artichoke, head

1 cup of cucumber, sliced

¼ tbsp of turmeric, ground

¼ tsp of cayenne pepper, ground

Preparation:

Wash the celery and chop into bite-sized pieces. Set aside.

Wash the cauliflower and trim off the outer leaves. Chop into small pieces and fill the measuring cup. Reserve the rest for later.

Wash the artichoke and trim off the outer leaves. Cut into small pieces and fill the measuring cup. Reserve the rest in the refrigerator.

Wash the cucumber and cut into thin slices. Fill the measuring cup and reserve the rest in the refrigerator.

Now, combine celery, cauliflower, artichoke and cucumber

in a juicer and process until juiced. Transfer to a serving glass and stir in the turmeric and cayenne pepper.

Serve immediately.

Nutrition information per serving: Kcal: 77, Protein: 8.3g, Carbs: 27.2g, Fats: 0.7g

18.   Sweet pepper Brussels Sprout Juice

Ingredients:

1 large sweet pepper, chopped

2 cups of spinach, chopped

1 cup of Brussels sprouts, chopped

1 large Granny Smith's apple, peeled and cored

¼ tsp of ginger, freshly ground

Preparation:

Wash the sweet pepper and cut lengthwise in half. Remove the stem and seeds. Cut into small pieces and set aside.

Wash the spinach thoroughly and torn with hands. Set aside.

Wash the Brussels sprouts and trim off the outer layers. Cut in half and set aside.

Wash the apple and remove the core. Cut into bite-sized pieces and set aside.

Now, combine sweet pepper, spinach, Brussels sprouts, and apple in a juicer.

Transfer to serving glasses and stir in the honey.

Add some ice and serve immediately.

Nutritional information per serving: Kcal: 196, Protein: 6.8g, Carbs: 55.6g, Fats: 1.4g

19.   Watermelon Apple Juice

Ingredients:

1 small wedge of watermelon

1 cup of pomegranate seeds

1 small green apple, cored

1 small ginger knob, sliced

1 oz of water

Preparation:

Cut the watermelon in half. Scrape out the seeds and cut one large wedge. Peel and chop into small pieces. Wrap the rest in a plastic foil and refrigerate for later.

Cut the top of the pomegranate fruit using a sharp paring knife. Slice down to each of the white membranes inside of the fruit. Pop the seeds into a measuring cup and set aside.

Wash the apple and cut lengthwise in half. Remove the core and cut into bite-sized pieces. Set aside.

Peel the ginger and cut into small pieces. Set aside.

Now, combine watermelon, pomegranate, apple, and

ginger in a juicer. Process until well juiced and transfer to a serving glass. Add some water to adjust the bitterness, if needed.

Refrigerate for 15 minutes before serving.

Nutrition information per serving: Kcal: 162, Protein: 3.1g, Carbs: 45.3g, Fats: 1.5g

20.   Butternut squash Lemon Juice

Ingredients:

1 cup of butternut squash, chunked

1 whole lemon, peeled

1 cup of fennel, chopped

1 cup of cucumber, sliced

Preparation:

Peel the butternut squash and remove the seeds using a spoon. Cut into small cubes and reserve the rest of the squash for some other recipe. Wrap in a plastic foil and refrigerate.

Peel the lemon and cut lengthwise in half. Set aside.

Trim off the outer wilted layers of the fennel. Roughly chop it and fill the measuring cup. Reserve the rest for later.

Wash the cucumber and cut into thin slices. Fill the measuring cup and reserve the rest in the refrigerator. Set aside.

Now, combine butternut squash, lemon, fennel, and cucumber in a juicer and process until well juiced. Transfer to a serving glass and add some crushed ice.

Serve immediately.

Nutrition information per serving: Kcal: 86, Protein: 3.4g, Carbs: 30.0g, Fats: 0.5g

21.   Grapefruit Parsley Juice

Ingredients:

1 whole grapefruit, peeled

2 cups of parsley, chopped

1 whole grapefruit, peeled

1 cup of watermelon, diced

7 oz of green beans, chopped

½ cup of pure coconut water

Preparation:

Peel the grapefruit and cut into small pieces. Set aside.

Wash the parsley under cold running water. Torn with hands and set aside.

Cut the watermelon lengthwise. For one cup, you will need about 1 large wedge. Peel and cut into chunks. Remove the seeds and set aside. Reserve the rest of the melon for some other juices.

Wash the green beans and chop into small pieces. Place them in a pot of boiling water and cook for 3 minutes. Remove from the heat and drain. Set aside.

Now, process, grapefruit, parsley, watermelon, and beans in a juicer.

Transfer to serving glasses and stir in the coconut water.

Add some ice and serve immediately.

Nutritional information per serving: Kcal: 161, Protein: 6.4g, Carbs: 45.6g, Fats: 1.5g

22. Artichoke Lemon Juice

Ingredients:

1 medium-sized artichoke, chopped

1 whole lemon, peeled

1 cup of whole cranberries

1 medium-sized apple, cored

¼ tsp of cinnamon, ground

Preparation:

Wash the artichoke and trim off the outer, hard leaves. Cut into bite-sized pieces and set aside.

Peel the lemon and cut lengthwise in half. Set aside.

Using a small colander, rinse well the cranberries. Drain and set aside.

Wash the apple and cut lengthwise in half. Remove the core and cut into bite-sized pieces. Set aside.

Now, combine artichoke, lemon, cranberries, and apple in a juicer and process until juiced. Transfer to a serving glass and stir in the cinnamon.

Refrigerate for 15 minutes before serving.

Nutrition information per serving: Kcal: 149, Protein: 5.9g, Carbs: 53.7g, Fats: 0.8g

23.   Apricot Oranges Juice

Ingredients:

2 whole apricots, pitted

2 large oranges, peeled

2 whole grapefruits, peeled

1 cup of collard greens, chopped

¼ tsp of turmeric, ground

Preparation:

Wash the apricots and cut lengthwise in half. Remove the pit and cut into bite-sized pieces. Set aside.

Peel the oranges and divide into wedges. Set aside.

Peel the grapefruits and divide into wedges. Cut each wedge in half and set aside.

Wash the collard greens thoroughly under cold running water. Drain and chop into small pieces. Set aside.

Now, combine apricots, oranges, grapefruit, and collard greens in a juicer and process until juiced. Transfer to a serving glass and stir in the turmeric.

Refrigerate for 10 minutes before serving.

Enjoy!

Nutrition information per serving: Kcal: 344, Protein: 9.3g, Carbs: 105.4g, Fats: 1.6g

24.   Blackberry Lemon Juice

Ingredients:

1 cup of blackberries

1 whole lemon, peeled

1 cup of beets, sliced

1 medium-sized pear, chopped

1 oz of water

Preparation:

Rinse well the blackberries using a small colander. Drain and set aside.

Peel the lemon and cut lengthwise in half. Set aside.

Wash the beets and trim off the green parts. Cut into thin slices and fill the measuring cup. Reserve the rest for later.

Wash the pear and cut in half. Remove the core and cut into bite-sized pieces. Set aside.

Now, combine blackberries, lemon, beets, and pear in a juicer and process until juiced. Transfer to a serving glass and stir in the water.

Refrigerate for 15 minutes before serving.

Enjoy!

Nutrition information per serving: Kcal: 165, Protein: 4.9g, Carbs: 60.2g, Fats: 1.4g

25. Watercress Sweet Pepper Juice

Ingredients:

1 cup of watercress, torn

1 large sweet pepper, chopped

1 medium whole tomato, chopped

1 rosemary sprig

1 oz of water

Preparation:

Wash the watercress thoroughly under cold running water. Slightly drain and torn with hands into small pieces. Set aside.

Wash the sweet pepper and cut lengthwise in half. Remove the stem and seeds. Cut into small pieces and set aside.

Wash the tomato and place in a small bowl. Chop into small pieces and make sure to reserve the tomato juice while cutting. Set aside.

Now, combine watercress, sweet pepper, and tomato, in a juicer and process until juiced. Transfer to a serving glass and stir in the water and reserved tomato juice. Sprinkle with rosemary and serve immediately.

Enjoy!

Nutrition information per serving: Kcal: 56, Protein: 3.5g, Carbs: 15.1g, Fats: 0.7g

26. Zucchini Cherries Juice

Ingredients:

1 medium-sized zucchini, chopped

1 cup of whole cherries

1 large wedge of honeydew melon

2 large strawberries

1 oz coconut water

Preparation:

Wash the zucchini and cut into thin slices. Fill the measuring cup and reserve the rest for later. Set aside.

Using a small colander, rinse well the cherries. Drain and set aside.

Cut melon lengthwise in half. Scoop out the seeds and then wash the melon. Cut one wedge and peel it. Cut into bite-sized pieces and set aside.

Wash the strawberries and remove the stems. Chop into small pieces and set aside.

Now, combine zucchini, cherries, melon, and strawberries in a juicer. Process until well juiced. Transfer to a serving glass and add few ice cubes.

Serve immediately.

Enjoy!

Nutrition information per serving: Kcal: 96, Protein: 1.8g, Carbs: 31.4g, Fats: 0.6g

27.   Swiss Chard Asparagus Juice

Ingredients:

1 cup of Swiss chard, torn

1 cup of asparagus, trimmed

1 large tomato, chopped

1 cup of Brussels sprouts, trimmed

1 large zucchini, sliced

Preparation:

Wash the Swiss chard thoroughly under cold running water. Drain and set aside.

Wash the asparagus and trim off the woody ends. Cut into 1-inch pieces and set aside.

Wash the tomato and place in a bowl. Cut into quarters and reserve the juice while cutting. Set aside.

Wash the Brussels sprouts and trim off the outer layers. Cut in half and set aside.

Wash the zucchini and cut into thick slices. Set aside.

Now, combine Swiss chard, asparagus, tomato, Brussels sprouts, and zucchini in a juicer and process until juiced.

Transfer to serving glasses and add some ice before serving.

Nutrition information per serving: Kcal: 109, Protein: 10.1g, Carbs: 32.4g, Fats: 1.2g

28.   Papaya Zucchini Juice

Ingredients:

1 cup of papaya, chopped

1 large zucchini, sliced

1 large tomato, chopped

1 large lemon, peeled

1 cup of fresh basil, chopped

Preparation:

Peel the papaya and cut lengthwise in half. Scoop out the black seeds and flesh using a spoon. Cut into small chunks and set aside.

Peel the zucchini and chop into small pieces. Set aside.

Wash the tomato and place in a bowl. Cut into quarters and reserve the juice while cutting. Set aside.

Peel the lemon and cut lengthwise in half. Set aside.

Wash the basil thoroughly and roughly chop it. Set aside.

Now, combine papaya, zucchini, tomato, lemon and basil in a juicer and process until juiced.

Transfer to serving glasses and add some ice before serving.

Enjoy!

Nutrition information per serving: Kcal: 240, Protein: 3.1g, Carbs: 75.1g, Fats: 0.9g

29. Coconut Pumpkin Juice

Ingredients:

1 cup of pumpkin, cubed

½ cup of coconut water, unsweetened

1 medium-sized banana, peeled

1 cup of raspberries, fresh

1 tsp of honey, raw

Preparation:

Cut the top of a pumpkin. Cut lengthwise in half and then scrape out the seeds. Cut one large wedge and peel it. Cut into small cubes and fill the measuring cup. Reserve the rest in the refrigerator.

Peel the banana and cut into chunks. Set aside.

Wash the raspberries under cold running water. Drain and set aside.

Now, combine pumpkin, banana, and raspberries in a juicer. Transfer to serving glasses and stir in the coconut water and honey.

Add some ice and serve immediately.

Enjoy!

Nutritional information per serving: Kcal: 153, Protein: 3.9g, Carbs: 49.1g, Fats: 1.3g

30.   Mixed Berry Coconut Juice

Ingredients:

1 cup of cranberries

1 cup of blackberries

1 cup of blueberries

1 cup of raspberries

3 oz of coconut water

Preparation:

Combine cranberries, blackberries, blueberries, and raspberries in a large colander. Rinse under cold running water and drain. Set aside.

Now, combine all in a juicer and process until juiced. Transfer to serving glasses and add some ice before serving. Optionally, add some honey for some extra taste.

Enjoy!

Nutrition information per serving: Kcal: 165, Protein: 5.0g, Carbs: 63.4g, Fats: 2.1g

31.   Lettuce Grapefruit Juice

Ingredients:

3 cups of red leaf lettuce, torn

1 large orange, peeled

1 large grapefruit, peeled

1 cup of papaya, chopped

½ cup of pure coconut water, unsweetened

1 tsp of liquid honey

Preparation:

Wash the lettuce thoroughly under cold running water. Torn with hands and set aside.

Peel the orange and divide into wedges. Set aside.

Wash the grapefruit and chop into small pieces. Set aside.

Peel the papaya and cut lengthwise in half. Scoop out the black seeds and flesh using a spoon. Cut into small chunks and set aside.

Now, combine lettuce, orange, grapefruit and papaya in a juicer and process until juiced.

Transfer to serving glasses and stir in the coconut water and honey.

Refrigerate for 10 minutes before serving.

Enjoy!

Nutrition information per serving: Kcal: 208, Protein: 4.3g, Carbs: 63.7g, Fats: 0.9g

32. Brussels Sprout Carrot Juice

Ingredients:

1 cup of cauliflower, chopped

1 cup of Brussels sprouts, chopped

1 cup of carrots, sliced

1 cup of turnip greens, chopped

3 large oranges, peeled

1 tbsp of honey

Preparation:

Trim off the outer leaves of a cauliflower. Wash it and fill and cut into small pieces. Fill the measuring cup and reserve the rest in the refrigerator.

Wash the Brussels sprouts and trim off the outer layers. Cut in half and set aside.

Wash the carrots and cut into thin slices. Set aside.

Wash the turnip greens thoroughly and torn with hands. Set aside.

Peel the oranges and divide into wedges. Set aside.

Now, combine cauliflower, Brussels sprouts, carrots, turnip greens, and oranges in a juicer and process until juiced. Transfer to serving glasses and stir in the honey and coconut water.

Add some ice cubes before serving or refrigerate for 10 minutes.

Enjoy!

Nutrition information per serving: Kcal: 367, Protein: 14.47g, Carbs: 116g, Fats: 1.9g

33.   Lemon Broccoli Juice

Ingredients:

2 large lemons, peeled

2 cups of raw broccoli, chopped

1 cup of fresh raspberries

½ cup of coconut water, unsweetened

2 large zucchinis, peeled and sliced

1 tbsp of honey

Preparation:

Peel the lemon and cut it lengthwise. Set aside.

Wash the broccoli and cut into small pieces. Set aside.

Wash the raspberries under cold running water. Drain and set aside.

Wash the zucchinis and cut into thick slices. Set aside.

Combine lemons, broccoli, raspberries, and zucchinis in a juicer and process until juiced. Transfer to serving glasses and stir in the coconut water and honey.

Add some ice and serve.

Enjoy!

Nutritional information per serving: Kcal: 192, Protein: 10.9g, Carbs: 56g, Fats: 2.2g

34.   Radish Asparagus Juice

Ingredients:

1 large honeydew melon wedge

1 large radish, chopped

1 cup of Swiss chard, torn

1 cup of asparagus, trimmed

1 cup of papaya, chopped

¼ cup of pure coconut water, unsweetened

Preparation:

Cut the honeydew melon lengthwise in half. Scoop out the seeds using a spoon. Cut the large wedges and peel them. Cut into small chunks and place in a bowl. Wrap the rest of the melon in a plastic foil and refrigerate.

Wash the radish and trim off the green parts. Cut into small pieces and set aside.

Wash the chard thoroughly and torn with hands. Set aside.

Wash the asparagus and trim off the woody ends. Chop into small pieces and set aside.

Peel the papaya and cut lengthwise in half. Scoop out the

black seeds and flesh using a spoon. Cut into small chunks and set aside.

Now, combine honeydew melon, radish, chard, asparagus, and papaya in a juicer and process until juiced.

Transfer to serving glasses and refrigerate 15 minutes before serving.

Enjoy!

Nutritional information per serving: Kcal: 127, Protein: 5.2g, Carbs: 37.0g, Fats: 0.8g

35. Swiss chard Guava Juice

Ingredients:

1 large guava, chopped

2 cups of Swiss chard, torn

2 cups of fresh kale, torn

A bunch of spinach, torn

¼ cup of pure coconut water, unsweetened

1 tbsp of pure coconut sugar

Preparation:

Wash the guava and cut into chunks. Set aside.

Combine Swiss chard, kale, and spinach in a colander and wash thoroughly under cold running water. Drain and torn with hands. Set aside.

Now, combine guava, Swiss chard, kale, and spinach in a juicer and process until juiced.

Transfer to serving glasses and stir in the coconut water and pure coconut sugar.

Add some ice and serve immediately.

Enjoy!

Nutrition information per serving: Kcal: 129, Protein: 48.1g, Carbs: 34.6g, Fats: 3.2g

36.   Grapefruit Orange Juice

Ingredients:

2 large oranges, peeled

1 medium-sized pear, roughly chopped

1 cup of spinach, torn

1 large grapefruit, peeled

1 small ginger root slice, peeled

Preparation:

Peel the oranges and divide into wedges. Set aside.

Wash the pear and remove the core. Cut into small pieces and set aside.

Wash the spinach thoroughly and torn with hands. Set aside.

Wash the grapefruit and chop into small pieces. Set aside

Peel the ginger slice and set aside.

Combine oranges, pear, spinach, grapefruit, and ginger in a juicer and process until juiced.

Transfer to serving glasses and refrigerate for 10 minutes

before serving.

Enjoy!

Nutritional information per serving: Kcal: 221, Protein: 5g, Carbs: 71.8g, Fats: 0.8g

37.   Coconut Lime Juice

Ingredients:

2 large limes, peeled

1 cup of broccoli, chopped

A bunch of fresh spinach

1 large grapefruit, peeled

1 cup of coconut water, unsweetened

1 tbsp of honey, raw

A few mint leaves

Preparation:

Peel the limes and cut them lengthwise in half. Set aside.

Wash the broccoli and trim off the outer leaves. Set aside.

Wash the spinach thoroughly and torn with hands. Set aside.

Wash the grapefruit and chop into small pieces. Set aside.

Now, combine limes, broccoli, spinach, and grapefruit in a juicer and process until juiced. Transfer to serving glasses and stir in the honey and garnish with mint leaves.

Add some ice and serve.

Enjoy!

Nutritional information per serving: Kcal: 176, Protein: 14.5g, Carbs: 52.0g, Fats: 2.07g

38.   Cherries Kiwi Juice

Ingredients:

1 cup of cherries

1 cup of cauliflower, chopped

1 cup of kale, torn

3 large kiwis, peeled

1 tsp of pure coconut sugar

Preparation:

Wash the cherries and remove the green stems, if any. Cut each cherry in half and fill the measuring cup. Set aside.

Trim off the outer leaves of a cauliflower. Wash it and fill and cut into small pieces. Fill the measuring cup and reserve the rest in the refrigerator.

Wash the kale thoroughly and torn with hands. Set aside.

Peel the kiwis and cut lengthwise in half. Set aside.

Now, combine cherries, cauliflower, kale, and kiwis in a juicer. Transfer to serving glasses and stir in the coconut water.

Add some ice and serve!

Enjoy!

Nutritional information per serving: Kcal: 228, Protein: 8.9g, Carbs: 66.2g, Fats: 2.3g

39.   Spinach Mixed Berry Juice

Ingredients:

1 cup of blueberries

1 cup of raspberries

1 cup of blackberries

1 cup of strawberries, chopped

¼ cup of spinach

½ tsp of ginger, ground

Preparation:

Wash the spinach thoroughly and torn with hands. Set aside.

Combine all berries in a colander and wash under cold running water. Set aside.

Now, mix all berries and spinach in a juicer and process until juiced. Transfer to serving glasses and stir in the ginger.

Add few ice cubes and serve immediately.

Enjoy!

Nutritional information per serving: Kcal: 158, Protein: 5.9g, Carbs: 56.4g, Fats: 2.3g

40.   Grapefruit Honey Juice

Ingredients:

1 large grapefruit, peeled

1 cup of pumpkin, cubed

2 large Granny Smith apples, cored and chopped

1 tsp of honey, raw

½ tsp of ginger, freshly ground

Preparation:

Wash the grapefruit and chop into small pieces. Set aside.

Cut the top of a pumpkin. Cut lengthwise in half and then scrape out the seeds. Cut one large wedge and peel it. Cut into small cubes and fill the measuring cup. Reserve the rest in the refrigerator.

Wash the apples and remove the core. Chop into bite-sized pieces and set aside.

Combine grapefruit, pumpkin and apples and process in a juicer. Transfer to serving glasses and stir in the honey and ginger.

Refrigerate or add some ice and serve.

Enjoy!

Nutritional information per serving: Kcal: 271, Protein: 4.5g, Carbs: 79.22g, Fats: 1.1g

41.   Cantaloupe Papaya Juice

Ingredients:

1 cup of cantaloupe, cubed

1 cup of papaya, chopped

½ cup of coconut water

1 cup of guava, chopped

1 tbsp of fresh mint leaves

¼ tsp of cinnamon, ground

Preparation:

Cut the cantaloupe in half. Scoop out the seeds and flesh. Cut and peel one large wedge. Chop into chunks and fill the measuring cup. Reserve the rest of the cantaloupe in a refrigerator.

Peel the papaya and cut lengthwise in half. Scoop out the black seeds and flesh using a spoon. Cut into small chunks and set aside.

Wash the guava and cut into pieces. If you are using large fruit, reserve the rest for some other recipe in a refrigerator.

Now, combine cantaloupe, papaya, and guava in a juicer.

Transfer to serving glasses and stir in the coconut water.

Garnish with some mint leaves and add some ice before serving.

Enjoy!

Nutritional information per serving: Kcal: 124, Protein: 3.3g, Carbs: 36.3g, Fats: 1.2g

42.   Strawberries Coconut Juice

Ingredients:

2 cups of strawberries, chopped

1 large red orange

1 cup of blueberries

½ cup of coconut water, unsweetened

1 tsp of pure coconut sugar

Preparation:

Combine blueberries and strawberries in a colander and wash under cold running water. Set aside.

Peel the orange and divide into wedges. Use about half of the wedges and reserve the rest for some other juice.

Combine blueberries, strawberries, and orange in a juicer. Transfer to serving glasses and stir in the coconut water and coconut sugar.

Add some ice or refrigerate before serving.

Enjoy!

Nutritional information per serving: Kcal: 146, Protein: 3.0g, Carbs: 45.8g, Fats: 0.8g

43.   Butternut Squash Cinnamon Juice

Ingredients:

1 cup of butternut squash, chunked

1 small pear, cored and chopped

½ tsp of cinnamon, freshly ground

¼ cup of water

Preparation:

Peel the butternut squash and remove the seeds using a spoon. Cut into small cubes and reserve the rest of the squash for some other recipe.

Wash the pear and remove the core. Cut into bite-sized pieces and set aside.

Wrap in a plastic foil and refrigerate.

Now, combine pumpkin and pear in a juicer and process until juiced.

Transfer to serving glasses and stir in the water and cinnamon.

Add some ice before serving and enjoy!

Nutritional information per serving: Kcal: 183, Protein: 3.4g, Carbs: 59.8g, Fats: 0.5g

44.   Carrot Apple Juice

Ingredients:

2 large carrots, sliced

1 cup of parsnip, sliced

3 Granny Smith's apples, cored and chopped

½ tsp of cinnamon, freshly ground

¼ tsp of ginger, ground

1 tbsp of honey, raw

Preparation:

Wash the carrots and parsnips and cut into thick slices. Set aside.

Wash the apples and remove the core. Cut into bite-sized pieces and set aside.

Combine carrots, parsnip, and apples in a juicer and process until juiced.

Transfer to serving glasses and stir in the honey, cinnamon, and ginger.

Add few ice cubes and serve immediately.

Enjoy!

Nutritional information per serving: Kcal: 406, Protein: 5.6g, Carbs: 121.8g, Fats: 1.9g

45. Zucchinis Grapefruit Juice

Ingredients:

3 large zucchinis, peeled

1 grapefruit, peeled

1 tsp of peppermint extract

1 oz of coconut water

1 tbsp of coconut sugar

Preparation:

Wash the zucchinis and cut into thick slices. Set aside.

Peel the grapefruit and cut into bite-sized pieces, set aside.

Now, combine zucchinis and grapefruit in a juicer and process until juiced. Transfer to serving glasses and stir in the coconut water, coconut sugar and peppermint extract.

Add some ice cubes and serve immediately.

Enjoy!

Nutritional information per serving: Kcal: 204, Protein: 7.7g, Carbs: 59g, Fats: 1.3g

46.   Celery Parsnip Juice

Ingredients:

1 cup of parsnips, chopped

2 large carrots, sliced

1 celery stalk, chopped

1 whole guava, chopped

2 large grapefruits, peeled

1 large orange, peeled

Preparation:

Wash the carrots and parsnips and cut into thick slices. Set aside.

Wash the celery and cut into small pieces. Set aside.

Wash the guava and cut into chunks. If you are using large fruit, reserve the rest for some other recipe in a refrigerator.

Peel the grapefruits and chop into bite-sized pieces.

Peel the oranges and divide into wedges. Set aside.

Now, combine parsnips, carrots, celery, guava, grapefruits,

and orange in a juicer and process until juiced.

Transfer to serving glasses and add some ice before serving.

Nutritional information per serving: Kcal: 328, Protein: 8.7g, Carbs: 101.2g, Fats: 2.0g

47.   Cantaloupe Juice with Fresh Peach

Ingredients:

1 cup of cantaloupe, diced

1 medium-sized peach, pitted

1 cup of mango, chunked

1 whole lime, peeled

1 cup of fresh mint, finely chopped

Preparation:

Cut the cantaloupe in half. Scoop out the seeds and cut two wedges and peel them. Chop into chunks and set aside. Reserve the rest of the cantaloupe in a refrigerator.

Wash the peach and cut lengthwise in half. Remove the pit and cut into bite-sized pieces. Set aside.

Wash and peel the mango. Cut into small chunks and set aside.

Peel the lime and cut lengthwise in half. Set aside.

Now, combine cantaloupe, mango, peach, lime, and mint in a juicer. Process until well juiced. Transfer to a serving glass and add some crushed ice.

Serve immediately.

Nutritional information per serving: Kcal: 205, Protein: 5.2g, Carbs: 59.2g, Fats: 1.6g

48.   Lime Cherry Juice

Ingredients:

1 cup of avocado, cubed

1 cup of fresh cherries, pitted

1 whole lime, peeled

1 medium-sized orange, wedged

1 tbsp of honey, raw

Preparation:

Peel the avocado and cut in half. Remove the pit and cut into small cubes. Fill the measuring cup and reserve the rest for later.

Wash the cherries and cut each in half. Remove the pits and set aside.

Peel the lime and cut lengthwise in half. Set aside.

Peel the orange and divide into wedges. Cut each wedge in half and set aside.

Now, combine avocado, cherries, lime, and orange in a juicer and process until well juiced. Transfer to a serving glass and stir in the honey.

Add some crushed ice and serve.

Nutritional information per serving: Kcal: 408, Protein: 6g, Carbs: 74.5g, Fats: 22.5g

49.   Raspberry Plum Juice

Ingredients:

1 cup of raspberries

2 whole plums, pitted

1 cup of apricots, sliced

1 medium-sized carrot, sliced

1 tbsp of honey, raw

Preparation:

Using a colander, wash the raspberries in under cold running water. Slightly drain and set aside.

Wash the plums and cut in half. Remove the pits and set aside.

Wash the apricots and cut lengthwise in half. Remove the pits and cut into thin slices. Fill the measuring cup and reserve the rest for later.

Wash and peel the carrot. Cut into thin slices and set aside.

Now, combine raspberries, apricots, carrot, and plums in a juicer and process until well juiced.

Transfer to a serving glass and stir in the honey. Add some

crushed ice before serving.

Nutritional information per serving: Kcal: 232, Protein: 5.3g, Carbs: 70.9g, Fats: 1.9g

50.   Cinnamon Kiwi Juice

Ingredients:

1 whole kiwi, sliced

1 cup of beets, sliced

1 small apple, cored

1 small pear, cored

¼ tsp of cinnamon, ground

Preparation:

Peel the kiwi and cut lengthwise in half. Set aside.

Wash the beets and trim off the green ends. Peel and cut into thin slices. Fill the measuring cup and reserve the rest for some other juice.

Wash the apple and pear. Remove the core and cut into bite-sized pieces. Set aside.

Now, combine beets, kiwi, apple, and pear in a juicer and process until well juiced. Transfer to a serving glass and stir in the cinnamon. Refrigerate for 15 minutes before serving.

Enjoy!

Nutritional information per serving: Kcal: 211, Protein: 4.2g, Carbs: 65.3g, Fats: 1.1g

ADDITIONAL TITLES FROM THIS AUTHOR

70 Effective Meal Recipes to Prevent and Solve Being Overweight: Burn Fat Fast by Using Proper Dieting and Smart Nutrition

By

Joe Correa CSN

48 Acne Solving Meal Recipes: The Fast and Natural Path to Fixing Your Acne Problems in Less Than 10 Days!

By

Joe Correa CSN

41 Alzheimer's Preventing Meal Recipes: Reduce or Eliminate Your Alzheimer's Condition in 30 Days or Less!

By

Joe Correa CSN

70 Effective Breast Cancer Meal Recipes: Prevent and Fight Breast Cancer with Smart Nutrition and Powerful Foods

By

Joe Correa CSN

www.ingramcontent.com/pod-product-compliance
Lightning Source LLC
Chambersburg PA
CBHW030245030426
42336CB00009B/266